Nature's Gifts
Healing and Relaxation through Aromatherapy, Herbs, and Tea

By Sheila M. Burke

Om Sweet Om Publishing

© 2014

Om Sweet Om Publishing

Printed and bound in the United States

Cover design by Sheila M. Burke © 2014

All rights reserved.
ISBN-13: 978-1500372255
ISBN-10: 1500372250
Library of Congress Card Number – Pending
ISBN-13: 978-1500372255
Nature's Gifts Healing and Relaxation through
Aromatherapy, Botanicals, and Tea   Om Sweet Om
Publishing

1st Edition

Contents

Botanicals – Historically Speaking

Since the prehistoric times, plants have been used and studied for use in medicine healing. In all times, cultures and civilizations (ancient and modern) plants have been known to treat ailments and illness. In fact, in modern times plants are studied and are the basis for many of our medications from pharmaceutical companies. They are even used in similar ways to treat things that once were treated by only the plant or derivative of the plant as it was applied traditionally, before we had pharmaceutical companies. Pharmaceutical companies use synthesized versions of these plants.

This is in part for two reasons. First, because plants generally cannot be patented by pharmaceutical companies, therefore a company cannot market the plant product as exclusive. Secondly, it is not easy to standardize or control the manufacturing of plants into medicine. (You don't know how much is in a product and it can vary from item to item.)

Did you know that out of the half million known plant species only about 5,000 of them have been studied for their medicinal values? Imagine all the knowledge out there just waiting to be discovered!

We have written record from the ancient Sumerians 5,000 years ago and all through the ages since then of the knowledge of healing and medicinal properties of herbs. From every corner of the Earth and every civilization including the Chinese, Romans, Greeks, Native Americans, Mayans, Egyptians, Hindus, the list goes on and on. Some of the earliest records are of course, the Sumerian tablets but there are also extensive records from 2500 B.C (Pen T'Shao Kang Mu: attributed to China's Yellow Emperor), 1550 B.C. (Ebers papyrus: Egyptian medical texts) and also an ancient Hindu scriptures which includes over a thousand plants used medicinally!

More recently we have the 1552 writings of Juan Badianus (a Native Mexican doctor) who recorded the widespread use of native herbs in medicine. The Europeans had what we call 'folk medicine' which is knowledge that's passed generationally by stories and tales at first, then by written word. Early American settlers brought their knowledge over and learned even more from the Native Americans about new species of plants. In the Middle Ages, monks recorded the knowledge of their time into extensive works incorporating their cultivating, planting, gardening and medicinal use of plants. And then we have who is now considered the first scientific botanist, Theophrastus who wrote the first 'true' herbal text that we know of called "De materia medica". In this text is listed over 500 medicinal plants studied scientifically. (Theophrastus 327-285B.C.) So this just goes to show you the historical use of botanicals in medicine and how we arrived at the place we are in today.

**Because botanicals can interfere with modern pharmaceuticals and cause interactions with them, you should always speak with your doctor before taking them! Also, very important: Before you ingest ANY herb or supplement, you need to educate yourself on the benefits as well as the downsides. If you have any sort of medical condition at all, you need to contact your doctor and discuss the herb with him because it may be harmful in your situation.

Botanical medicine is a major part of many traditional therapies. For instance, Homeopathy, Aromatherapy, Traditional Chinese Medicine, Shamanic Medicine and Ayurvedic Medicine to name a few. Botanicals are substances obtained from plants. Examples include fresh or dried materials and essential oils. Botanists estimate that there are over 250,000 species of flowering plants on the Earth. Three quarters of the Earth's population rely on herbal or botanical medicine*. *World Health Organization estimate.

Homeopathy – What Is It?

The philosophy of homeopathy: *"Like Cures Like"*. The belief that disease and illness is caused by a disturbance in the 'life force' or 'vital force'.

Homeopathy was founded by Samuel Hahnemann in the 18th Century. (Although Hahnemann gave the world the name 'homeopathy', this has been practiced for thousands of years before him)

What is it? Well, it's the belief that by diluting a substance so much, until there are no molecules remain for use in treating disease and illness. Most laws do not govern homeopathic remedies like they do for 'conventional treatments', therefore some question the effectiveness and safety of these treatments.

Hahnemann's homeopathy incorporated his belief that all illness had spiritual causes as well as physical. He also believed that you need to change your lifestyle to what we would call 'living healthy', such as exercising, eating healthy, and taking good care of your body.

In 1805 and 1810 he published "Materia Medica Pura" and "The Organon of the Healing Art" (which is still used by homopaths today). They documented his research known as 'proving'. Proving was his testing of what effects certain substances produced in people. He would have a person ingest a certain substance. By having them record all symptoms and really, everything they felt and experienced which taking a substance, he could learn how to treat like diseases. And because he found that using large doses of a substance caused worsened illness, he advocated extreme diluting of those substances.

One widely known experiment that he conducted was that he himself ingested large amounts of cinchona bark (which was a known cure for Malaria) to see if he could produce the symptoms of Malaria. He did. Understanding that the cure for Malaria also produced symptoms for Malaria, became his starting point for 'like cures like' and his homeopathy.

Considering that medicine during his time consisted of bloodletting and leeches, and concoctions that included everything from opium and snake venom, heavy use of laxatives and things we would consider today to be insane - homeopathy really took off back then and by 1900 there were homeopathic colleges and practitioners throughout the world. In the United States alone, there were 22 established colleges and over 15,000 practicing Homeopaths. By the 1950's there were less than 100 still practicing pure homeopathy in the US, but it seems it may be making a comeback once again.

*Note: To give you but one example of homeopathy today: A 200C dilution of duck liver, sold under the name "Oscillococcinum" is a popular treatment for the flu!

Coconut! For a Healthy
Inside *and* Outside!

Coconut oil has been used for thousands of years for nutritional and health benefits as well as skin care. It comes from the meat or kernel of a mature coconut.

The oil is comprised mainly of saturated fatty acids (nearly 94%) and very rich in Lauric Acid and Vitamin E and K and Iron. Unlike other saturated fats, it is broken down quickly and turns into quick energy for the body. Because it does this, it is not stored like other saturated fats in the body. The benefits of ingesting coconut oil are far reaching and I'll touch on them a bit: Very effective against infection. Coconut oil is a terrific immune booster because it's packed with lauric, caprylic and capric acids and lipids!

A wonderful, natural antiviral & antifungal as well as being antibacterial. Great to fight against yeast infections, diaper rash and, athlete's foot.

Tackles and kills bacterias that cause UTI's, ulcers and infections of the throat.

Coconut oil helps to control blood sugar and helps insulin secretion. Wonderful for your kidneys and beneficial to your liver. Great for your bones! Coconut helps the body absorb many minerals including calcium – so it's great for our bones and teeth.

Now on to skin care!

Coconut oil is amazing for the skin! Often compared to mineral oil, it is SO beneficial! But, unlike mineral oil, there are no adverse side effects to the skin (unless of course you are allergic to it.)

Great for people suffering from dermatitis, eczema, psoriasis as well as those with dry skin.

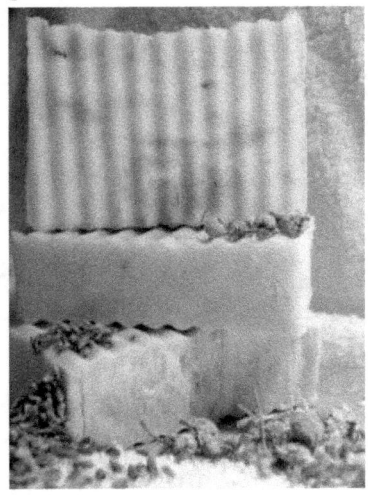

A wonderful acne treatment due to its high content of lauric and capric acids. When you rub coconut oil on your skin, microbes on the skin take these acids and turn them into monocaprin and monolaurin. This process converts or replaces the protective layer of acid on your skin. This combined with the high content of Vitamin E (which we know keeps our skin healthy and happy) is a wonderful combination. That Vitamin E will help to make sure your sebum glands are healthy and clear.

Coconut oil is also very well absorbed into the skin and helps to keep it more elastic. A great natural treatment for rashes and superficial wounds. Beautiful free radical fighter! The more antioxidants we have on our skin and in our body's tissues and cells, the better we are in our ability to fight those nasty free radicals. And a direct result of this would be smooth, supple, soft skin.

Use it to condition your scalp and hair! Not only a superb dandruff fighter, but a shine builder, follicle penetrating dryness preventer! (When using it on the hair, you should apply it, let it sit a bit (even overnight if you want to), and then shampoo it off).

How's that for an all-around skin care product? And best of all *it is natural.*

The Many Benefits of Rosemary

Rosmarinus Officinalis, or Rosemary, is a member of the mint family. Rosemary is known widely as an herb

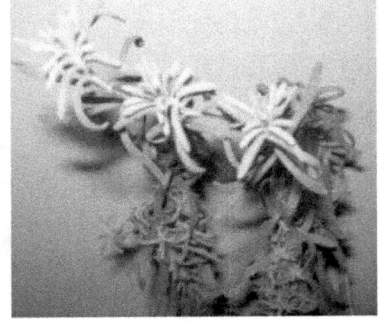

used in cooking. But did you know that since ancient times, it has been used to benefit the human body in many, many more ways?

Rosemary essential oil is extracted from the leaves of the plant. Because the oil is a natural antiseptic, anti-fungal and antibacterial there are many wonderful ways in which you can incorporate Rosemary into your skin and body care.

When used on the skin in soaps, lotions and bath products, Rosemary will help tone your skin and retain

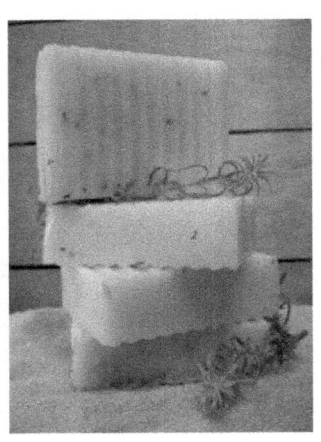

your natural moisture. It smells great by itself but can be combined with other essential oils and botanicals to tantalize your senses and give you a truly relaxing and beautifying feeling. Rosemary is known to stimulate the brain!

The aroma is a great addition to any students' study corner because it stimulates brain activity and makes you feel alive and awake. Put a couple drops in a diffuser or in a bowl of steaming water and just inhale it's wonderful aroma. You can even put a few drops into a spritzer bottle to keep handy and give your surroundings a bit of a spritz!

If you do not have rosemary oil, get a rosemary plant and pluck off some leaves to make potpourri. Used as a pain reliever in a rub or bath water is great for skin conditions, arthritis and rheumatism, sore muscles and even headaches! Used on the face it is a natural acne treatment.

When added to shampoos, rosemary oil will tingle your follicles and strengthen them! It's wonderful for dry scalp and getting rid of pesky dandruff! Massage a bit of oil onto the scalp and give your head a wonderful treat!

I keep a rosemary plant on my window sill to clip leaves and season foods like chicken, lamb and pork. This is nothing new of course, but did you know that rosemary leaves when chewed are great for gas, indigestion, stomach cramps and upset stomach?

Women can also benefit by chewing rosemary leaves when experiencing PMS, cramps and uncomfortable bladder.

Chewing the leaves will not only alleviate a sour stomach, but will freshen your breath as well! It is even said to help with sore gums and gingivitis pain.

There are also many household uses for rosemary oil! If you place a few drops onto a cotton ball and hang it in a closet, it will repel moths. Concoct your own disinfectant with rosemary oil in water, or simply use as a potpourri.

Peppermint – So Many Benefits!

Peppermint oil has a strong menthol aroma that is 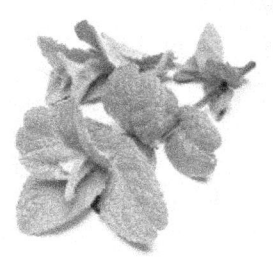 incredibly refreshing and stimulating. The benefits of peppermint have been touted for thousands of years.

Originally coming from the Mediterranean, it's now widely grown and harvested in many countries including the US and Great Britain.

The mints have been known for their analgesic, antiseptic and astringent qualities, but did you know they are great decongestants and expectorants as well? Remember when you had a stomach ache your grandmother gave you some hard peppermint candy to suck on? That's because it soothes the achy tummy as well! You can also use it to alleviate stress!

Peppermint is great because it is beneficial in so many forms and through so many senses! You can rub it on your gums for toothaches and sore gums, you can drink the tea or use candy to sooth your tummy or cramps, and it's great for colic and opens the nasal passages and sinus cavities!

The smell benefits asthmatics and those with chest congestion and in the bath or shower - peppermint (and spearmint!) are wonderful for relaxing sore muscles and achy feet!

Peppermint oil is packed with minerals, nutrients and vitamins like A and C. It also has omega 3 fatty acids that good for the body! Peppermint has actually gone through rigorous testing and IS proven effective!

*On a fun note: The name peppermint comes from Greek mythology. Minthe was loved and adored by Pluto (and underworld god). But, Pluto was already married and his wife was very very jealous of Minthe. So jealous that she in fact turned poor Minthe into a plant. Devastated, Pluto couldn't reverse the deed, but gave this new plant a beautifully powerful aroma so that he could enjoy her beauty even from afar.

**WARNING! Never use mint oils/products if you are allergic to menthol! And since peppermint is antispasmodic, you should avoid using during pregnancy. Never put it in your eyes! I've also seen recommendations to consult your doctor for use in children 8 and under.

Aloe Vera (Great Inside *and* Out!)

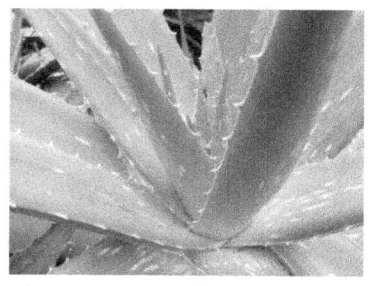

(Aloe barbadensis)

This plant belongs to the Asphodelaceae family. It is related to asparagus and onion plants. We find reference in ancient records to aloe vera and its benefits as far back as Dioscorides in 10 BC. Cleopatra (the ancient beauty queen) circa 50BC and even in Egyptian burial rituals.

The aloe vera plant is packed full with Vitamins A, B12 and E...and minerals including calcium, magnesium, and zinc which promote the healthy functioning of the body. And yes, this means you can ingest it! (The juice). When used externally aloe vera will help speed up the natural healing process of the body.

Aloe soothes the digestive system by telling your body to release pepsin. Pepsin is made by our bodies through our gastric system. It is an enzyme that is required to digest our food.) It's also an anti-inflammatory and anti-bacterial which could help explain why it helps those with ulcers, colitis and other stomach and bowel ailments.

Aloe juice is also used for bladder infections, kidney infections, heartburn, keeping the liver healthy, stimulation of the immune system with increased white blood cell production (to fight those nasty germs and viruses), arthritis, asthma, cramps in the legs, constipation and so much more!

When applied to the skin it can alleviate itching and soothe rashes and bumps. Just crack open a thick part of the left, give it a squeeze and let that sweet gel cover the area in question. It can be directly applied to a burn or superficial cut. *See a doctor for severe burns!

A great application for scars, fever blisters, cold sores, insect bites and dry skin. A wonderful natural moisturizer! In the mid 90's they started testing aloe vera for use in HIV treatments and it's also said to have benefits for those with diabetes.

Take chilled aloe vera gel, mix with a tiny bit of water and honey and you have a sweet, healthy snack!

*MEDICAL WARNING: Consult your doctor if you are using oral corticosteroids. If diarrhea or cramping develops stop ingesting!

Always do a small patch test before using a new product to see if you are allergic.

The Rose – Centuries of Beauty

The Rose has much to offer your skin! Rose water can be made at home by fashioning your own "still," but I would recommend buying it. The only thing to make sure of, is to look for 100% natural rose water on the label.   (Many products contain synthetic rose oil or water which, if you want this for therapeutic purposes or for use on your skin you do NOT want synthetic because it will not benefit your skin in any way. You must get natural.)

100% natural rose water is slightly astringent and has anti-bacterial properties. Many people use this to treat acne because it is very gentle on skin. Everyone should have a spritzer bottle handy filled with rose water. Use it before putting on your make up (helps to lay your foundation evenly) and when taking it off (helps to remove makeup so you don't have to rough up your face removing makeup).   Rose water helps to even out skin tone, restore moisture and even calm down swollen capillaries that make your face look all red and blotchy. It's also been known to soothe infections of the eye.

Men and woman both should use this as an aftershave splash! Rose water is such an all-around must have for all skin types! Whether you need to balance, tone, cleanse, cool, soothe - rose water is great for all these needs!

When looking for a good foundation, make sure natural rose extract is listed in the ingredients. Rose extract (again, natural!) helps to even your skin tone, give you a glow, hydrate and even soften your skin.

Rose Hip Oil is very rich in fatty acids, minerals and vitamins and is an anti-oxidant. This is why it is a key ingredient to good skin health. It has been said for many, many years that this oil gives a boost to your body's collagen and elastin levels because of its natural tretinoin derived from Vitamin A).

Finely ground Rose Hips are a wonderfully beautiful addition to skin cleansers as a natural exfoliate!

Rose Essential Oils are beautiful in aromatherapy! Put a drop or two into a diffuser or even a bowl of steaming hot water. Inhale that beautiful soothing aroma and relax!

Did you know that the rose is considered a type of mild natural sedative? Many people use it to relieve stress, tension and to calm nerves.

Drinking Rose Hip Tea will help maintain good digestion, secretion of bile and even help the circulatory system. It will also soothe a sore throat, calm diarrhea and give some relief to bladder infections.

Rose Hips are extremely rich in Vitamins A, B3, C, D and E, citric acid, flavonoids, bioflavonoids, tannins and zinc. Use roses in bath tea or facial steams, essential oils, a spray spritzer, tea or in any form, but make sure you incorporate the rose into your beauty regimen!

Cucumber Spritzer and the Benefits of Cucumber

Cucumbers are an awesome source of Vitamins C and A (A is mostly in the peel). And rich in folate, phosphorus, sodium, Vitamin B, potassium, sulfur, silica, calcium and manganese! They are roughly 95% water!

Here's a very cool all-purpose spritzer you can make in a matter of minutes at home! It's great any time of day, safe for your skin and it's natural!

In a blender, liquefy 1 cup of water and a half a cucumber (sliced up first). *Leave the peel ON, because it's packed with Vitamin A! Strain the mixture through a cheese cloth, twice. (You can also use a coffee filter) – Make sure you get all the pulp/lumps out so that it's only liquid. Pour it into a spray bottle and spritz away! (Keep in fridge up to one week)

You can spritz your face, hair, body and even the air! It's a wonderful pick-me-up and wonderful for your skin and hair!

DID YOU KNOW?

When you EAT a cucumber you are deriving all these benefits:

Cucumber juice, because of its acidity, helps regulate the body's blood pH therefore neutralizing acidity.

Regulates blood pressure (due to its contents of minerals and sodium)

Connective tissues, building: The excellent source of silica contributes to the proper construction of connective tissues in our body as in the bones, muscles, cartilage, ligaments and tendons.

Cucumber and celery blended together and made into a juice will help regulate your body temperature. Great to drink when you have a fever! The juice is also a soothing treatment for gastric and duodenal ulcers.

Cucumber juice is used to dissolve kidney stones and it makes you urinate. A wonderful natural diuretic. High in electrolytes and will re-hydrate the cells within your body.

Great for inflammation in many parts of the body, including the one part we think of most often regarding puffiness - the eyes (one slice each eye for 10-15 minutes)

Contains silicon and sulfur which is great for promoting hair growth.

The high amount of vitamin C and anti-oxidants makes it a wonderful natural treatment for skin problems like eczema, psoriasis, acne, rashes, bug bites, and sunburn! Now go eat a half a cucumber and make yourself a spritz with the other half!

Chamomile. It's As Good As Your Grandmother Said!

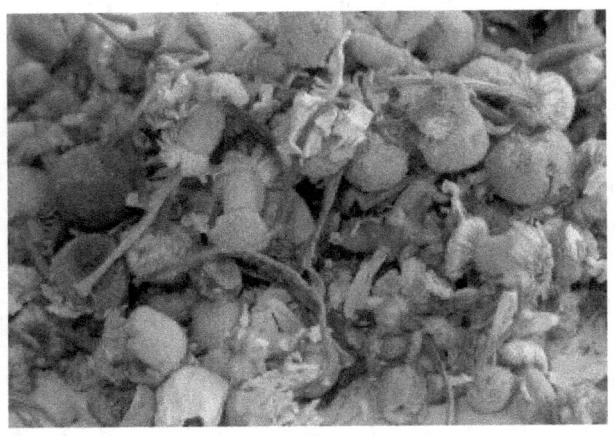

Matricaria recutita (German variety of chamomile)
Chamaemelum nobilis (Roman variety of chamomile
The German variety is found most often in the US. The Roman, in the UK.

Chamomile has long been known for its healing qualities both internally and externally. But why? Chamomile flowers contain volatile oils (favonoids and essential oils). Essential oils soothe the skin and tissue and actually help irritated skin. These essential oils are often used to help heal bug bites, stings, burns and even acne. Essential oils from chamomile flowers contain including bisabolol, bisabolol oxides A and B, and matricin. Flavonoids (namely 'apinegin' in chamomile) are anti-oxidants that help the body's natural healing process and combat free radicals. Chamomile acts like a natural stress reliever and sedative because it relaxes the muscles in the brain. Chamomile is beneficial to children as well as adults. Which is nice because natural treatments for children are often times limited. It's very beneficial for teething pain and colic spasms in babies. And provides a natural calming and soothing feeling as well. Chamomile is anti-allergenic, anti-spasmatic, anti-fungal, anti-pyretic, anti-peptic, antiseptic and anti-bacterial.

All those little stories that your grandmother passed down about Chamomile are indeed true. From calming the nerves, soothing sore muscles and PMS, relaxing after a long day, soothing a stomach ache - chamomile is a wonderfully natural way to go! Drink two or three cups of chamomile tea daily and you'll feel better. You can also soak in a warm bath of chamomile and breathe in its healing goodness! The subtle scent will work on your olfactory senses and relax your brain and body. You can also put chamomile in facial steams and grains.

Here's a short list of how chamomile can help your body. You'll be amazed!

Sleep Aid

Stress Relief

Nausea

Gets your bowels moving

Aids in digestion

Relieves colds, flu and sinus issues

Relieves Allergies

Morning Sickness

Teething

PMS

Cramps

Sore Muscle Relief

Gastritis

Hemorrhoids

IBS

Heartburn

Peptic Ulcers

Gas

Ulcerative Colitis

Crohn's Disease

Colic

Diverticulitis

Skin Irritations (eczema, psoriasis, bites, minor burns, ulcers, rashes, wounds)

Conjunctivitis

Eye Inflammation

Sunburn

Mouth Sores and Gum Disease (use as a mouth wash)

Recipe for chamomile tea:

Boil water to a rolling boil then remove from heat.
Put 1/8 cup or a couple tablespoons dried chamomile
flowers into the pot. (About 2 teaspoons per 8 oz. cup)
Let the pot steep for 15-20 minutes.
Drink.

*Note: You can also use the above recipe for a foot bath,
mouth wash, gargle, or to soak clean dressings for mild
burns.

*Also note: Although chamomile creams are wonderful,
you should never use this on a burn, as often times
creams contain oily ingredients that actually trap the
heat in the skin and making you feel worse. Mild burns
should be treated with chamomile tea (must be cooled)
applied to a clean dressing.

Honey and Skin Care

Honey attracts and retains moisture. In order for our skin to stay elastic, soft and supple it has to retain moisture.

Over time (aging) our skin loses that elasticity and ability to retain moisture, thus we get wrinkles.

Our skin needs antioxidants, plain and simple. These protect our skin from the sun and help to rejuvenate aging cells. Honey is packed with antioxidants and naturally hydrates. Honey will give your skin deep nourishment. It is also antiseptic and antimicrobial which means it wards off some bacterias. All these wonderful qualities of honey make it an exceptionally great natural facial product. Honey is wonderful for acne and for all skin types including sensitive!

Honey recipes:

Face Mask

In a bowl using a whisk, combine 1 egg white and 1 1/2 tablespoons honey (support your local honey growers). Combine this with enough clay to form a paste. (You can use flower but clay is preferred.) Leave on 5-15 minutes depending on your skin type – longer for oily) Wash off gently with warm water and pat dry.

Hair/Scalp Conditioner

Combine 2 Tablespoons of olive, sunflower, virgin coconut or hemp oil and 1/2 cup of honey. Massage it into your scalp and let sit for 20-30 minutes. Wrap hair in a towel. If you do not have this much time, do this while in the shower. Put the mixture in your hair and leave it sit while you are washing your body. Rinse thoroughly and shampoo lightly afterwards.

Acne

Wash your face with a warm saline solution (water and a little salt). With a Q-Tip, dab natural honey on your pimples and leave it sit on there for five to ten minutes. Rinse with warm water and gently pat dry.

Combine 1/4 cup natural honey, 1/2 teaspoon of real lemon juice, 2 Tablespoons yogurt and 2 pureed strawberries. Mix well. Wash your face with the mixture and rinse well with warm water. Pat dry.

Lavender for the Whole Self!

Lavender is great for your physical and mental wellbeing!

What is actually in lavender?

The aroma comes from the aldehydes in lavender. These also contribute to the soothing effects of the flower.

Lavender also is full of ester. Esters are known to boost and balance your mood and help with depression. They

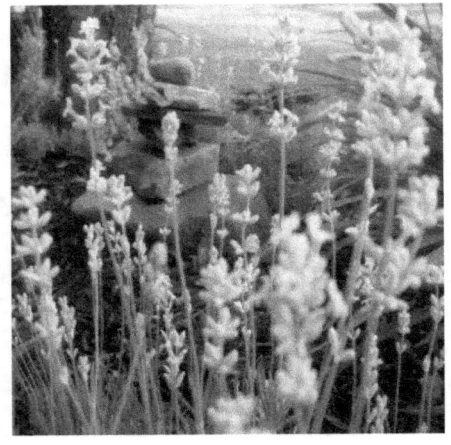

calm swelling and help lessen scarring. They will also help calm muscle spasms!

Lavender also has ketones which are known analgesics, and they help reduce swelling and build healthy tissue. They also make people sleepy.

Linalol kills bacteria and virus germs and lavender has a lot of it!

Lavender (unlike many other essential oils) CAN be directly applied to the skin. A little bit is great for sunburns! Simply add a few drops to a spray bottle of water, and mist away! Have a mosquito bite? Dab a bit of lavender on it! Remember, it has anti-itching properties!

*notes: pregnant women or those with serious medical conditions (i.e. diabetes) should not use lavender.

What specifically is lavender good for?

Lavender is great for relaxation and for calming your nerves! Put a few drops on a small pillow at bedtime and let yourself sink into a wonderful nights sleep! Or put a few drops in a warm bath and relax for twenty minutes. (Mix with sea salts and you've got one delicious spa bath!) You can even massage a drop or two into your temples gently to relieve stress and tension!

You can use lavender to relieve PMS! Since it is loaded with anti-inflammatories (natural anti-inflammatories) this is a beautiful addition to your stock of natural remedies! Massage the lower part of your back and abdomen with a couple drops of lavender essential oil, or as above use in the bath. The scent and feel of lavender will help you relax, ease tense muscles and balance the mind.

Did you know you can use lavender to help your acne, skin and even your hair? Yes! With a Q-Tip, dab your pimples with a bit of lavender essential oil (2x

daily).   For your hair, you can add 5-10 drops of lavender essential oil and the juice of one fresh lemon to a quart or so of mineral water (distilled or spring will also work well).   After washing and rinsing your hair, massage your lavender/lemon juice mixture into your hair, put it up in a towel and leave for thirty minutes. (A great time to read a book or give yourself a facial!) Better yet, treat yourself to a lavender facial!
**Great for getting rid of dandruff!

Freshen up with lavender!
Clip some fresh lavender, dry it out for a week or so by rolling it tightly in newspaper, and when dry break it up and put it into little sachets to freshen up underwear drawers, linen cabinets - anywhere that can use some lavender love!
Calm your stomach and nerves!
Use a heaping tablespoon of dried (or fresh) flowers into a pot of boiling water. Remove from the heat and let steep ten minutes or so. Strain and sip.

*note - pregnant women should NOT use lavender (nor those with serious medical conditions! Always consult your doctor when using herbs!)

Okay so what if I don't have time to do any of this?

If a little stress relief on the go is what you're looking for simply pinch off a sprig of lavender, gently rub it in your fingers back and forth. The smell will remain for a while. Just breathe in the beauty of what lavender has to offer you!

Garlic! Wonderful Garlic!

The National Academy of Sciences states that eating garlic boosts our natural supply of hydrogen sulfide which acts as an antioxidant and sends signals in our cells to relax our blood vessels and increase the flow of blood.

Way back to the time of the ancients, garlic has had known medicinal properties. And through research in modern times we're learning the ancients were (big surprise) right all along! By eating garlic and thus giving your body the ability to ramp up its production of hydrogen sulfide you are protecting your heart and giving a big boost to your immune system. Garlic helps make the platelets sticky which helps reduce blood coagulation.

Studies say two or three cloves a day (cook it into your food) reduced subsequent heart attacks in people who have had them by fifty percent. Studies are also finding there is a correlation between people who have a garlic rich diet have some sort of protection against certain cancers like colon, breast, prostate, stomach, liver and lung. Garlic contains more than thirty anticancer compounds and antioxidants. The most powerful are allin, ajoene, quercetin, nitrosamine and aflatoxin. Apparently, according to these studies, ajoene and allicin have been found to be like a natural chemotherapy to cancer cells. Another benefit of garlic is it helps regulate the body's blood pressure. So whether you have problems with low or high blood pressure, garlic can help equalize it. Garlic is stuffed full with vitamins and nutrients including Vitamins A, B, B2 and C, Calcium, Zinc, protein, potassium, and the minerals selenium and manganese.

Garlic helps to strengthen your body's natural defenses against allergies and colds. It's a wonderful natural expectorant and decongestant and can even help protect the body from bacteria and viruses. Chop up three or four cloves and put it in soup to relieve a cold or flu.

It helps loosen plaque from artery walls, regulates blood sugar levels and blood pressure (whether your pressure is high or low, it will help balance it). Garlic makes your body produce nitric oxide in the walls of your blood vessels which helps you relax. There are many homeopathic remedies using garlic. From ringworm to warts, toothaches to tonsillitis, ear infections to sore throats and sinus infections, asthma to herpes. You can take garlic in a pill form also (available at health food stores). Although I think they are still studying the effects of pill form garlic in comparison to actually ingesting it.

Special notes!

Garlic (and onions) are toxic to cats and dogs.

Garlic thins the blood similar to the effect of an aspirin.

To get rid of the garlic smell on your breath (ewe) eat a couple lemon wedges.

Don't eat garlic before surgery or delivering a baby. (It thins your blood)

Don't eat garlic if you have a blood disorder.

Don't eat it in excess! A clove or two daily should be sufficient.

Oatmeal. Not Just for Breakfast Anymore.

When using oatmeal in skin care, do not get quick oats. Use only rolled oats. Plain ol' rolled oats with nothing else at all added. The oatmeal recipes for skin care use ground rolled oats. Simply put a scoop in the blender and grind it into a fine powder. (The consistency of flour)

Not only is oatmeal wonderful for your insides, it's wonderful for your skin as well! A great natural exfoliate, oatmeal will cleanse away the dirt while invigorating the top layer of the skin and removing dead skin cells. A great natural cleanser, oatmeal will leave your skin clean, smooth, supple and elastic!

Oatmeal has been used for thousands of years to relieve bug stings, bites, dryness, itchy skin, chickenpox, eczema, sunburn and many types of sensitivities.

Packed full of wonderful natural properties your skin needs and enjoys, oatmeal leaves a protective barrier on your skin and is a natural moisturizer!

Body Scrub Recipes

These are very easy and can be done in your own kitchen! Make them in small amounts so they are always fresh and bacteria free. Don't keep them longer than a couple of weeks.

Brown Sugar Oatmeal Body Scrub

2 Tablespoons brown sugar (can use white)
6 Tablespoons ground rolled oats (in blender)
6 Tablespoons pure honey (support your local grower)
1 1/2 teaspoons pure lemon juice or fresh squeezed.
Combine all ingredients in a bowl, mixing well until reaching a paste like consistency. Wet your skin and gently apply the mixture. The length that you leave it on your skin is up to you but generally 3-5 minutes is good! Rinse well with warm water.

Face & Body Scrub

1/4 C ground rolled oats
2 Tablespoons fresh lemon juice
Enough olive oil, aloe vera juice, yogurt or milk to make a paste.
Mix all together into a workable paste. Spread over the areas you wish to cover. Let sit 3-10 minutes and wash off thoroughly with warm water. Pat lightly with a clean soft towel.

Bath Treat

Use the above recipe only scoop the mixture into a muslin bag and toss in the bath as the water is running. Throw some salts into the bag for added skin benefits!

Ripe Banana Facial Mask

1/4 of a mushy (very ripe but not rotten!) banana
2 Tablespoons natural clay or flour
1/8 teaspoon ground cinnamon
2 Tablespoons ground rolled oats

Carefully add a little milk but just enough to get the mixture into a smooth paste. If you add too much milk, just throw in a bit more oats, clay or flour.
Smooth on to dampened skin and let sit for 3-10 minutes depending on your skin type (dry skin 5 minutes, oily 10 minutes, and sensitive 3 minutes)
Rinse well with warm water and splash with cool water. Pat dry with a soft clean towel.

Astragalus – More Than Just an Ancient Root.

Also known by: milk vetch, huang qi, huang ch', radix astragali, goat's horn, green dragon, and locoweed.

Scientific/medical name: *Astragalus membranaceus*

For more than 2,000 years, Chinese herbalists have recommended astragalus root to build energy and the immune system. The most commonly used herb in China today, it is said that astragalus helps to resist diverse diseases including cancer, heart disease, liver and kidney problems, and infections. Studies by the American Cancer Society, the National Cancer Institute, as well as five other cancer institutes, indicate that astragalus actually helps build the immune system during chemotherapy. (It is not a CURE for cancer! It has NOT been found to attack cancer cells!)

What is it commonly used for?
Strengthens the immune system

Improves digestion

Gives you energy and endurance

It's an antibacterial

Improves white blood count

Prevention of heart disease

Treatment of fibromyalgia

Treatment of diabetes

Stimulates the spleen, liver urinary and circulatory systems

Lowers blood sugar and blood pressure

Treatment of arthritis

Is there evidence that it works?

YES! And, it's scientific evidence! Astragalus enhances the immune system and fights diseases, including cancer and heart disease, and colds and flu! Researchers at The Anderson Cancer Center (U of TX) found that astragalus extract enhanced the cell-destroying ability of the conventional immunotherapy treatment interleukin-2 by improving the immune system's response. They also tested it in test tubes, and found that it partly restored the immune function of cells. It also stimulates the production of interferons, (produced by the body as part of the normal defense mechanism) against colds, sinusitis, flu, upper respiratory, and viral infections.

In 2006 there was a review of the most reliable studies of the root pertaining to lung cancers. Evidence was found that astragalus enhances the effects of some chemotherapy drugs and boosted the immune system in cancer patients.

Are there any possible problems or complications?

(From the American Cancer Society):

Astragalus is generally considered safe. Reported side effects include abdominal bloating, loose stools, low blood pressure, and dehydration. People with autoimmune diseases (such as rheumatoid arthritis or lupus) or people taking immune suppressing medicines (such as corticosteroids or cyclosporin) should talk to their doctors before taking this herb. There is some concern that astragalus might interfere with blood clotting, so some doctors recommend it should not be taken before surgery or in people taking aspirin-like drugs or blood-thinning medicines. It may also affect blood pressure in some, so those taking blood pressure medicines may need to be monitored by their physicians. There have also been reports of lowered blood sugar, which could be dangerous for those with diabetes or hypoglycemia.

Don't use if you have an immune system disease like MS, Lupus or Rheumatoid Arthritis or anything considered an autoimmune disease.

Don't use if you are pregnant or nursing.

Always check with your doctor before using herbs/supplements and with your pharmacist if you are taking any medications.

How can you take it?

You can boil four ounces of the whole root in a quart of water for 10 minutes, let steep, strain and drink as tea. (2-4 cups a day) *don't take the tea if you have a fever. Swallow it in pill form available at your local health food store.

Hemp! Great for the Skin and So Much More!

Okay, let's get the *one misconception* about hemp out of the way from the start. Hemp oil is the result of pressing the seeds of the cannabis salva plant and *it cannot get you high*. It does not contain THC.

With that said, let's explore the wonderful benefits of hemp!

Hemp seed and oil are loaded with natural goodness for your body! Highly rich in essential omega 6 and 3 fatty acids, amino acids and Vitamin E that your body craves and needs! Seventy to eighty percent of the seed contains these Omega's!

When eaten, the omega 3 fatty acids are a wonderful natural anti-inflammatory and are a tremendous benefits to those suffering from chronic joint pain and arthritis. A great addition to any diet! Helps prevent heart disease, controls blood pressure, increases energy, controls high cholesterol, promotes healthy development of the brain and nurtures and protects the hair, scalp and skin!

Hemp oil is also mineral rich including calcium, magnesium, phosphorus, potassium and sulfur. It will also supply you with a healthy dose of carotene and chlorophyll.

Specifically relating to skin care, hemp oil is an all-around benefit. People suffering from eczema, psoriasis, scaly or dry, cracked, damaged or irritated skin will find relief in hemp oil, as will those who have had laser treatments and sunburn. It's also wonderful for use on the lips!

The Omega 6 and Lineolic Acid in hemp oil help to keep water and moisture in your skin. As nature's moisturizer, the oil helps to create a barrier between your skin and the harsh air around you. That air contains pathogens, viruses, bacteria and all kinds of gross chemicals that will cling to your skin. It is also great for treating acne because it combats the bacteria on your skin. Hemp will also bring those weakened lipids in your skin back to life and bring a little more bounce back into aged skin.

Hemp Seed Oil has the highest ratio of Omega 6 to Omega 3 fatty acids than all the other oils. It has the least amount of the *bad* fats (saturated and mono-unsaturated) and is valuable both when ingested and applied to the skin.

If you are cooking with hemp oil, keep in mind that heating it over 150 degrees is not good for the human diet. In fact, it is not recommended for consumption over 150 degrees. ***Cook on low heat only***.

It is best when used in place of other oils for salad dressing, tossing spaghetti noodles, adding to drinks (like a smoothie or milkshake), or add to things like sauces and soup. (It's a great substitute for olive oil, flax seed and fish oil – although all these oils are wonderful for us as well!)

HEMP SMOOTHIE

1 cup fresh cut up strawberries

1 banana

1 apple cored, stemmed and cut

2 cups orange or pineapple juice

2 scoops hemp protein powder (health food store)

1 and 1/2 Tablespoons hemp seed oil

1 and 1/2 cup ice cubes

Blend in a blender until smooth. Great for adults *and* kids! Wonderful summertime treat!

Aromatherapy: Air Freshening, Facial Steams, and Facial Teas

A Brief History

Aromatherapy uses essential oils and other aromatic compounds found in plants, to cause an effect on a person's mind or body. This has been used for thousands and thousands of years. All ancient civilizations used scents for bathing, massage and embalming.   Aromatherapy shows the distinctive properties used to heal which are obtained from pure essential oils. The make-up of the molecules in the oils allows the chemical in the oil to penetrate the tissue in the body and move very rapidly to the limbic system. The limbic system is a part of the brain structure of all mammals associated with olfaction, autonomic functions and certain areas of emotion and behavior.

Certain scents are known to trigger responses or reactions within human bodies. For instance, your grandmother wore gardenia, so when you smell gardenia, you may remember the warmth of her touch and the comfort of her smile. This causes you to be relaxed and alert. When you are relaxed and alert, you feel better, you can manage pain better, you can think better and you are less stressed.

Although this has been used for thousands of years, if we go back to 1564, we find an alchemist named Giovanni Battista della Porta. He recorded methods used to separate essential oils from the distilled waters that were widely used in the millenia prior. In 1937, Rene-Maurice Gattefosse (a French chemist) developed what is known as Modern Aromatherapy.

Now first of all, you cannot just go and grow stuff in your back yard and expect to practice real aromatherapy. The quality and chemical make-up of the herbs depend greatly on the cultivation and care of the herbs while growing. There is a ton of research involved as well as knowledge of horticulture. Much care needs to be given to the plants, the timing, harvesting, storage, weather, soil conditions, etc.

Air Freshening

Aromatherapy uses essential oils and other aromatic compounds found in plants, to cause an effect on a person's mind or body. This has been used for thousands and thousands of years. All ancient civilizations used scents for bathing, massage and embalming. Certain scents are known to trigger responses or reactions within human bodies. For instance, your grandmother wore gardenia, so when you smell gardenia, you may remember the warmth of her touch and the comfort of her smile. This causes you to be relaxed and alert. When you are relaxed and alert, you feel better, you can manage pain better, you can think better and you are less stressed. Freshen the air you breathe with essential oils! Simply put a couple drops of essential oil or an essential old blend into a bowl of hot water. *Keep up and out of the reach of children and pets.* (You can also put the bowl on a table and drape a towel over your head, and let it steam your skin – *this is called a facial steam or facial tea*). Alternatively you can put the drops into a vaporizer, a diffuser, a humidifier, spray bottles (diluted with water), dishes and even hot candle wax!

There are many blends for a variety of results! Here are a few of my favorites:

CLEAN FRESH SCENT:
Pine – 2 drops
Cedarwood – 2 drops
Vanilla – 1 drop

SLEEP/RELAX:
Chamomile – 3 drops
Lavender – 3 drops

LOVE/ROMANCE:
Ylang Ylang – 2 drops
Orange – 1 drop
Geranium – 1 drop

LOVE/ROMANCE:
Jasmine – 2 drops
Rose – 1 drop
Ylang Ylang – 1 drop

CELEBRATION:
Lemon – 1 drop
Lime – 1 drop
Bergamot – 2 drops
Cedarwood – 2 drops

MOTIVATION:
Bergamot – 3 drops
Ginger – 2 drops
Balsam of Peru – 4 drops

COZY/WARMTH:
Cinnamon – 2 drops
Clove – 1 drop
Apple – 3 drops

THANKS/GRATITUDE:
Sandalwood – 3 drops
Pine – 1 drop
Rose – 1 drop

REJUVENATE:
Juniper – 3 drops
Lemongrass – 3 drops
Lemon – 2 drops

AWARENESS:
Rosemary – 2 drops
Eucalyptus – 2 drops
Tangerine or Orange – 2 drops
Peppermint – 1 drop

*Generally, scents are not recommended if you or someone in your home/space has asthma!

Steams and Teas for the Face (All Natural and Organic)

Any of the combinations of scents above can be used as a facial steam or facial tea. A facial *steam* is a bowl of hot water with the herbs or scents in the water. Sit with the bowl on a sturdy surface such as a table, and put your face over the bowl (approximately 12 inches away) with a towel draped over your head and the bowl. Natural & Organic Herbal Steam Spa for your face!

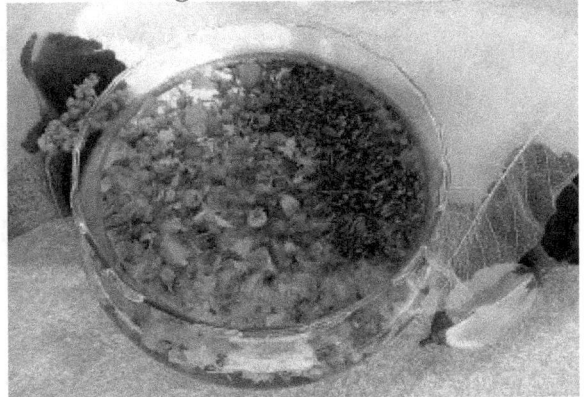

The ultimate in multi-tasking! Open your pores, say goodbye to flaky dead skin cells and toxins! Deep clean - all while sitting, relaxing and breathing in healthy, beautiful aroma!

You can make your own facial steams, or facial teas, but please be careful when purchasing your herbs. You want to make sure you are buying certified organics and make sure the process the grower uses for drying will be such as your herbs do not contain bacteria.

Chamomile is very beneficial to our bodies. The active ingredients found in the chamomile flower are volatile oils (aka essential oils and flavonoids). Essential oils are known to soothe the skin and have been proven to help irritations of the skin. Flavonoids are anti-oxidants and protect your body from harmful free radicals. They help your body to heal. Chamomile is also calming to the nerves and very relaxing.

Rose Hips when used externally (in this case, the oils from the hips) has wonderful regeneration properties and will aid with the feelings of stress and that overall feeling of being worn-out. Very relaxing and calming.

Peppermint contains an amazing, natural therapeutic ingredient called menthol. This will give you a cool, relaxing feeling. The aroma will revitalize your senses and put a little spring into your day!

Cinnamon is a wonderful stress reducer! Filling the air with the scent of cinnamon will calm your nerves. The smell of cinnamon essential oils are known to boost your memory.

Lemongrass acts like an astringent, opening pores and refreshing the skin!

Calendula flowers, bright yellow and orange and packed with natural skin benefits! There is a huge difference between Marigolds you grow in your flowerbed and organic Calendula flowers which are native to the Mediterranean.

Calendula contains flavonoids which we already know are very beneficial to our body. The flower of the Calendula has anti-inflammatory, anti-fungal, antiseptic and astringent properties. For millenia people have been applying Calendula to the skin when they suffer from rashes, bug bites, sunburn, windburn, itchy skin and scalp, boils and other skin irritations. Calendula from the Mediterranean should never be confused with your garden variety Marigold.

Make your own facial steam

3 cups water (distilled is best, but tap is ok)

One rounded 1/4 measuring cup dried herbs

Bring water to a boil in a non-metallic pan

Reduce to a simmer, add herbs, COVER, and continue to simmer 1-2 minutes remove from heat and let steep 1-2 minutes. (During this time, you should wash your face with water. It is best to use steam facial on clean skin)

Set the pan in an area where you can sit comfortably in front of it. Cover the back of your head with a clean towel and bring the ends of the towel around the pan (to capture the steam, like a First, make sure the steam is not too hot. It should feel comfortable. Keep your face within 8-12 inches from the steaming pan. Keep your eyes closed, listen to quiet music or just relax. Breathe normally but deeply through your nose. Keep your face in the steam a few minutes, then back up a bit as to cool your face. Do this for 10-15 minutes.

*Note: An alternative to sitting over the pot, is to soak a clean washcloth in the pot. (Make sure temperature is not too hot!) Wring out the cloth and apply to your face for a few minutes. Take off and repeat several times.

Follow up with a clay facial mask or gently pat face with witch hazel or cold water.

**Do not ingest. ***Do not reuse steamed portion. Discard used portion into garden or compost.

Natural Remedies for Colds

What better way to learn about alternative treatments then to look toward the very people that survived on this land without any modern knowledge of medicine. Native Americans never took more than they could use and always replenished what they did take. If they killed a buffalo, they used every bit of it for something, including the skin and bones. If they picked a plant, they only took as much as they needed.

And I got to thinking, these people, just like the ancient cultures in Asia, survived for thousands of years on what nature provided. Everything had a use. In fact, most of our medicines today are derived from the same herbs and plants that the natives used.

Let's look at cold remedies:

Echinacea builds the immune system. It's not going to cure the cold, but it lessons it and helps your body fight it. I remember years and years ago when this first came out, the FDA said, "Oh, that's not safe, "Oh, it's not regulated." *Now it's in everything.*

Goldenseal: This works to promote a healthy spleen. Spleens produce white blood cells to fight viruses.

Garlic: It can actually block the cold virus! Although it's said that garlic is most effective when eaten raw, it can also be made into tea (smash a few cloves in one cup of water and let steep six hours, strain and drink) Also, when you eat garlic, the active ingredients shoot right to your respiratory system!

Willow Bark: First off, don't give this to children. It has salicin in it, which is like Aspirin. Very, VERY bad for kids, but adults can take it to fight fevers, aches and pains. Willow Bark Tea: 1 teaspoon to 1 Cup boiling water. Let steep 15 minutes, strain and drink.

Licorice: No, I don't think Twizzlers qualify here. The Native Americans used real licorice to clear out the lungs. It's an expectorant! And it's also helpful in treating stomach ulcers, colic and inflammation. It also increases the body's interferon which helps fight viruses. Drink it in a tea: Mix 1 teaspoon of licorice syrup to a cup of boiled water. Note: Pregnant woman should never take licorice. And no one should overdo it when ingesting it because you can get high blood pressure.

Ginger: Not only does ginger reduce fever but it relieves pain, headache and motion sickness, and it helps to stop the cold virus in its tracks. You can buy ginger at the grocery store. It's an ugly rooty looking thing. Look for a smooth brown skin on the bulb, it should be hard and heavy. Chop fresh ginger and steep a teaspoon full in a cup of boiling water.

Note: Ginger is also used for athlete's foot! Cool the tea and soak your feet in it. Since ginger contains *cineole* it helps with stress relief and boosts your mood. You can even drink ginger ale, just make sure that you look at the ingredients: must say made with real ginger. If it doesn't contain real ginger, you'll just get a sugar rush, and be more stressed.

**If you are pregnant or nursing or on any other medicines, you should never ever take herbals without asking your doctor. Never.

**This is not intended to be medical advice. Always consult a doctor when ill.

How to Fix Dry, Cracked Skin

If you're like most of us on the planet, you suffer from dry, itchy skin during winter months. Dry, itchy skin is caused by many things including cold, wind, smoke, chemicals in soaps and poor diet (deficiencies of vitamins A and B). It can also be caused by medical conditions such as diabetes, under active thyroid, dermatitis, eczema, psoriasis and seborrhea.

So what do we do? The following is a list of great do-it-yourself options:

Avoid high alkaline laundry soap and body soap.

Use soap that is a neutral ph. A great choice would be a goatsmilk soap. Goat's milk is closest to human ph than any other! *Avoid commercial soaps that are not natural or that contain detergents! They will deplete your natural oils!

When you wash your face, do not use a washcloth. It can be too abrasive on dry, chapped skin. Instead, wash by splashing MINERAL water (NOT tap as tap water will dry it even more) and then gently blotting dry with a clean soft towel. *You can also fill a clean misting or sprayer bottle with mineral water (add a drop of lavender if you wish!) and mist your face during the daytime. Lightly blot your face dry after wards.

Use a humidifier. If you don't have one, put small bowls of water in front of heating vents.

When bathing or showing do not use very hot water. It will dry you out even more.

Do NOT use products that contain hydrogenated oils! Not only are they bad for your insides when you eat them they are bad for your skin. Use only products that contain pure oils such as olive, avocado, almond and sesame. Moisturize with natural shea butter or cocoa butter. Goatsmilk and yogurt are also wonderful for our skin!

Stay OUT of the wind and sun as much as possible.

Drink a lot of water and eat foods rich in essential fatty acids! Drink herbal teas such as chamomile, dandelion, peppermint or calendula. These are all wonderful for the skin!

Use facial steams! You can use any of the teas above as a facial steam! Steams are beautiful treats for your face and can be done right in your own home any time of the day.

For dry cracked hands/fingers try calendula cream, vitamin E, and aloe vera. Mix into a paste and apply it to the hands at bedtime. Leave a thin film if your hands are really cracked and dry, and put gloves on over the mixture for when you are asleep.

Use all natural facial grains every 3 days or a natural dry clay mask once weekly. You can mix some green or kaolin clay with honey to make your own. To make your own simple recipe without clay try mashing a banana with a little milk or mash up a bit of avocado with a teaspoon of lime juice. (*Clay is beneficial because it contains nutrients for your skin. Clay will not dry you out, it will actually help pull out the bad stuff in your skin, while putting moisture in.)

Take a milk bath! Ahhhh, these are wonderful treats for your skin! There is no limit to how often you can indulge yourself with one of these wondrous remedies! To make your own, you'll need powdered milk (goats milk or coconut is best, but whole milk or powdered will be okay), a natural oil like olive or almond and a few drops of essential oils like chamomile or lavender. As you are running your warm bath water, just drop these ingredients in, get in the tub and relax for 15-20 minutes! (You might want to kill two birds with one stone and do your grains or clay mask at the same time!) *Instead of oils you can use Dead Sea salts which in and of themselves are packed with vitamins and minerals for your skin!

Eat foods high in sulfur like eggs, asparagus, garlic and onion! (Garlic can also be taken in pill form to boost your immune system!)

Eat your fruits and veggies! Especially the yellow and orange ones! These are high in beta-carotene. Make sure you include seeds and nuts into your diet too. Avoid fried foods, alcohol, caffeine, and hydrogenated oils in your diet.

Use a couple drops of one of these essential oils in your bath, spray bottle or one drop with pure olive or almond oil on your skin:

Calendula

Chamomile

Geranium

Lavender

Patchouli

Rose

Sandalwood

Ylang-Ylang

You can also make your own massage oils with the essential oils above.

And finally, get a good nights sleep! Your cells repair themselves while you are sleeping!

All About Tea

What's in it, Benefits, Preparation, and Types

I am a tea lover. I love everything about it – the taste, the smell, and the sight of it! There is really much more to tea then steeping a bag in hot water. From health benefits to where tea comes from and everything in between, there is a lot to learn about tea. First we'll start with where tea comes from, then we'll look at what is in tea that is so good for us, and finally well look at the types of tea and its specific benefits and preparations.

Although there are many varieties of tea, there is only one plant that produces real tea. This is the evergreen shrub known as Camellia sinensis. By "real" tea I mean the four basic types of tea: white, black, green and oolong. These real teas are also the only teas that contain polyphenols. (Because they are grown from the Camellia sinensis bush) These teas are different are as a result of the process in which they are harvested.

Polyphenols have a strong taste to them. Black tea has only half the amount of polyphenol content than green teas, which may be the reason that black tea is one of the most consumed.

Green teas are becoming increasingly popular due to recent studies on their cancer fighting properties.

Green teas also contain the unique amino acid theanine as well as tannins, lignin, organic acids, proteins, sugar and caffeine. Theanine has been shown in research to be able to cross the blood-brain barrier. This means that it has psychoactive abilities which can cause temporary changes in brain function including perception, behavior and mood. Tests have also shown that theanine reduces stress levels and when ingested along with caffeine can improve mood and cognitive performance. The only other known source of Theanine, at this time, is from a certain mushroom.

Tannins have astringent like qualities as they are able to constrict tissues for example, around the intestinal tract, reducing diarrhea. They also will help in the same way as a gargle for sore throats. As with any medical condition, always consult a doctor before using anything for medicinal purposes, especially if you are taking medications and if you have a diagnosed condition. For instance, you will not want to use tannins to treat diarrhea if you have an intestinal or gastrointestinal disease or chronic problem.

Flavonoids are a subclass of polyphenols. Flavonoids protect the body from diseases by protecting the membranes of cells. They are thought to play a role in preventing hardening in the arteries, preventing stroke, heart disease and cancers. Flavonoids are found in almost every vegetable and fruit. They are found to be in very high levels in red wine, cooked tomatoes, berries, cabbage, broccoli, cauliflower, turnips, apples, onions and tea. White and green teas have exceptionally high amounts of flavonoids. And green tea also has a natural detoxification effect on the body. Herbal teas are wonderfully beneficial as well! Making "teas" out of dried (or fresh) flowers leaves, seeds, and herbs are not true teas, rather they are infusions - or more specifically - tisanes. Since herbal infusions are not really tea and not made from the tea bush, they do not contain caffeine.

TYPES OF TEA – How to prepare and what it does for the body

* **Please Note**:   Information on usage is based on traditional and/or folklore medicinal uses or stories that claim natural materials support health. This information has not been evaluated or approved by the FDA and is not necessarily based on scientific evidence from any source. These statements have not been evaluated by the Food and Drug Administration (FDA). These recipes are not intended to treat, diagnose, mitigate, prevent, or cure any condition or disease. If conditions persist, please seek advice from your medical

doctor. And always seek the advice of your doctor when taking medicines for possible interaction with any ingredient listed here.

Acerola Cherry Tea - Second only to Rose Hips in the amount of Vitamin C contained within. Also an excellent source of Vitamin A. Acerola Cherry is a number of antioxidants and fights free radicals and toxins. Contains thiamin, riboflavin, niacin, iron, calcium, phosphorous and potassium.

Helps heal wounds and scar tissue. Considered antibacterial, anti-fungal and anti-inflammatory. Said to help mastitis (breast pain), body cleansing, fever, diarrhea, colds/flu, infections, scurvy, stomach aches, hepatitis, digestive issues, dysentery, post menopause and preventing tooth decay.

Usually found as a blend in tea bags. Taste=Fruity

Allspice Tea - Use for relaxation and to uplift the mood. Provides relief from the common cold and upset stomachs. It has anesthetic qualities and is also said to prevent allergies, help with gas, bloat and burping and lower blood sugars. Many use it for muscle and joint pain. Allspice actually comes from the dried, unripened fruit of the pimenta dioica plant (native to Jamaica, West Indies, Central America and Mexico). It tastes like a combination of cinnamon, cloves, nutmeg and juniper. To make the tea, take 1 or 2 teaspoons of the powder (or the fruit) and put it into a cup of boiling water. Steep 15-20 minutes. (Strain if using the fruit)

Angelica Tea - Important notes: Do NOT use Angelica during pregnancy. Also: can cause sensitivity to light.

Angelica is related to the carrot, fennel and dill plants. This tea may improve digestion, hacking cough, blood circulation, PMS, gas, UTIs, tense intestinal muscles and sore gums. May also be useful as a compress for boils.

Put 1 teaspoon dried root into a cup, then fill with boiling water. Steep 10 minutes and then strain.

Anise Tea – Has a licorice taste. Good for coughs (loosens phlegm), gas, colic and nausea. Also great for colds, sinusitis and lung problems such as pneumonia and bronchitis.

1 teaspoon dried leaves (3 teaspoons fresh, crushed leaves) to 1 cup boiling water. Steep 5 minutes. Strain.
*Note: too much can cause a narcotic effect, so easy on the anise.

Bearberry (Uva Ursi) Tea - Made from the leaves which are picked in autumn and heat dried. Native Americans would drink the teas to help back sprains. Bearberry leaves also are a powerful astringent and is said to help bladder and kidney infections. Taste = Bitter. Pour 1 cup boiling water over two teaspoons dried leaves (or use infusion ball) and steep 10 minutes. Strain.

Blackberry Tea – 1-2 teaspoons of leaves per cup of hot water. Steep 10 minutes with an infuser ball. Good for diarrhea, sore throat, as a compress for varicose veins and hemorrhoids (good astringent). It is said to be a good complement to preventing cancer and heart disease.

Black Cohosh - Important note: Do not use black cohosh if you are pregnant! Rich in Vitamins A and B5 black cohosh also contains acctaeine, glcosides, estongenic sterols, isoferulic acid, oleic acid, palmitic acid, phosphorus, racemosin, tannins and triterpenes. Native Americans are among those ancients that have utilized this herb widely. It is known to balance hormones because it contains a natural estrogen. Helps menstrual cramps and uterine cramps. Cohosh has solicylates (anti-inflammatories) which calm the nervous system. It's said to be good for arthritis, sciatica, muscle pain and cramps, sinusitis, hot flashes, high blood pressure and maybe even asthma.

Blessed Thistle Tea – (originally named for its supernatural healing powers) An antimicrobial used for hundreds of years for a number of ailments including increasing mothers milk, a healthy digestive system, a healthy liver and gallbladder, making the heart and lungs stronger and improved memory (thistle increases oxygen content in the body). Also reduces fever and quiets chronic headaches. Treats infections. *Monks grew blessed thistle as a cure for small pox.

Taste- Bitter (can be mixed with mint, spearmint, or chamomile)

For tea: Put 1/2 oz. of dried blessed thistle into 1 cup boiling water. Steep 10-12 minutes. Can drink 3x daily. *Do not ingest if allergic to plants in the daisy family. *Can cause nausea and vomiting if too strong.

Blood Root Tea – Important note: Do NOT use during pregnancy! Also, may cause nausea and vomiting.

Pour 1 cup boiling water over 1/2 teaspoon of the dried root (cut/sifted). Cover and steep 3-5 minutes. Strain.

*Bloodroot is a protected plant. You cannot pick from the wild. Do not handle fresh plants without gloves.

Boneset Tea – Said to help upper respiratory infections and calm muscle aches during bouts of the flu. Pour 1 cup boiling water over 1 teaspoon of the dried boneset herb. Cover and steep 3-5 minutes. Strain.

Bugleweed Tea - A flowering plant in the mint family. Contains glycosides, tannins, organic acids and volatile oils. Said to calm the nerves like a mild sedation. May help in suppression of coughs, fighting tuberculosis, calming the heart rate, helping circulation and getting rid of excess fluid. Helps cyclic breast pain and moderates estrogen levels. Although studies show that it might be helpful in treating hyperthyroidism you should always talk to your own doctor first before using bugleweed.

For tea: 1 teaspoon dried bugleweed in an infuser ball. Fill cup with boiling water. Steep 10-15 minutes. Can take 3x daily.

Burdock Tea – Important note: Do NOT use during pregnancy or in children under 2 years old. Burdock root has high amounts of insulin and mucilage. The root can actually be chewed. (Roots should be picked in the fall, when they are two years old) Because of the high amount of insulin in the root, there may be value in it for diabetics. Burdock also stimulates the immune system, controls blood sugar, helps joint pain, abscesses, infections that are respiratory in nature, improves the lymph circulation, removes toxins from the skin, helps boils and skin sores, eczema and psoriasis and even cleans the blood. (And externally you can apply it to wounds, eczema, psoriasis and pimples) Mix 1 teaspoon of burdock root into 1 cup boiling water. Steep 10-15 minutes. Strain. *If mixed with Dandelion, this is good for liver detox. *If mixed with yellow dock and sarsaparilla, this is good for skin conditions.

Calendula Tea- Said to help many skin disorders including shingles and eczema and soothes stomach ailments such as ulcers, inflammation, gastritis and ulcerative colitis. It also relieves menstrual cramping, sore throats and inflammation of the mouth. Stimulates the production of collagen. Detoxifying.

When the calendula oil is used externally it can help relieve earaches. Tea washes may help conjunctivitis of the eye, acne, shingles, inflamed skin, eczema and hemorrhoids. Calendula is very high in flavonoids which make it a great anti-inflammatory and beneficial in many ways.

For tea: Put 1-2 teaspoons of calendula flowers in a cup or infuser ball and let steep 15 minutes in boiled water. Can be taken 3x daily.

Catnip Tea - Important note: Do NOT use during pregnancy! Said to work wonders on colds/flu, upset stomach, coughs. Fever reducer. Used also as a relaxer. Use a tea infuser. Put 1 teaspoon catnip leaf/flower into 1 cup boiling water. Cover. Steep 3-5 minutes.

Chai Tea – (Chai is Chinese for tea). There are many unique recipes for Chai. Mostly they contain black tea mixed with a variety of spices such as anise, cardamom pods, ginger, cloves, cinnamon, vanilla, pepper, nutmeg and more. The ancient Indians mixed certain spices with the tea to calm the mind and renew the spirit. There are many different recipes but my personal favorite is black tea (in a tea bag), a pinch of fresh ginger, a shake of cinnamon (or a few scrapes of a cinnamon stick), 2 inches of a piece of vanilla bean. Bring a cup and a half of water to a boil and add ingredients. Simmer 5-7 minutes. Then add a tablespoon of honey and teaspoon of sugar and 1 1/2 cups of milk. Bring to a boil, remove from heat and strain well. Serve hot or cold. For a quick pre-mixed chai, my absolute favorite is Oregon Chai Tea Mix in Original flavor. **See also: entry for **Masala Chai**

Chamomile Tea – Important note: Do NOT drink chamomile tea if you are pregnant! This tea has been used since ancient times for many varieties of conditions. Chamomile is known to produce glycine (an amino acid) in the body, which helps relieve muscle spasms and is a nerve relaxer. Many women drink the tea to relieve menstrual cramps because it's known to relax the uterus (which is why you shouldn't drink the tea if pregnant). Chamomile can also make you sleepy and soothe your stomach.

Don't boil the water with the flowers in it. Instead, pour a cup of boiling water over 1Tablespoon of chamomile flowers and let steep for 5 minutes. Strain if not using a tea ball. Additionally, you can mash up a slice of apple and put it in with the flowers when steeping.

Chickweed Tea – Important note: Do NOT use if pregnant or if you have existing medical conditions unless you consult your doctor.

Very high in potassium, magnesium, calcium and Vitamin C. For many years it is been appreciated for its treatment of skin and stomach problems. Can be ingested and used topically. Use for detoxification or to suppress the appetite. Beneficial for treatment of acne, rashes, boils and burns. It has been said that chickweed may help dissolve the plaque inside blood vessels, clean the blood and may help stop stomach or bowel bleeding and cleans the intestinal tract. When applied topically it can be used to acne, eczema, torn ligaments and swelling. (Dip cotton ball into warm tea and apply – or use spent tea bags)

For drinking: brew fresh or dried plants. Boil cold water in a pot. Let 1 tablespoon steep for 5 minutes in an infuser ball. Add honey or milk to improve taste. Serve hot or cold.

Chrysanthemum Tea – Taste = Sweet. Fever reducer. Neutralizes toxins and helps protect from liver damage. Said to be good for sinus congestion, clean the blood, lower blood pressure, cooling the body during sunstroke and relieves symptoms of colds/flu. Also said to sharpen the mind, vision and hearing.

Wash and drain 10-20 chrysanthemum flowers. Pour 3 cups water over them. Let steep 5 minutes. Strain.

Cinnamon Tea - Calming. Good for digestion, upset stomach, colds and circulation. Said to lower cholesterol and blood sugar.

Put a stick of cinnamon into a cup of boiling water, cover and steep 5-8 minutes. Add regular tea (in a teabag) and steep 1-2 minutes more. Sweeten if needed.

Clove Tea – Said to clean out and disinfect the bronchial membrane.

Colon Cleansers - these act like a laxative and is also used in detoxification. Use only occasionally! (Can cause nausea, diarrhea and cramping)
Types of Colon Cleansing teas: Rhamnus purshiana bark, berberis vugaris bark, cassia senna leaves, and capsicum frutescens.

Damiana Tea - Said to help menstrual cramping, ease depression. Stimulant, Diuretic.
Pour 1 cup boiling water over 1 teaspoon of damiana herb (dry). Cover and steep 3-5 minutes.

Dandelion Tea - Contains more beta-carotene than carrots! Leaves contain Vitamins: B1, B2, B5, B6, B12, C, D, E and P; and iron, zinc, phosphorus, magnesium, potassium and calcium. Harvest the leaves before the flowers come out in the spring or wait until after the first frost in autumn. Five to six leaves (torn into strips) will make one cup of tea. Place the leaves in the bottom of the cup and pour boiling water in. Let that stand 10 minutes then strain. It is very bitter by nature. You can drink sweetened with honey or sugar or unsweetened. Unsweetened can also be applied to the skin as a cleaner. *You should not use dandelion if you have a bowel or bile duct obstruction or problems with the gallbladder.

Dill Tea - Good for upset stomachs, colds, flu, fever, bronchitis, UTIs, insomnia, and may aid in digestion. Calms the nerves and cleans the blood.
Crush dill seeds (or grind). Add 1 teaspoon of crushed seeds into 1 cup of boiling water. Steep 3-5 minutes and strain.

Echinacea Tea - Best known for its immune system boosting abilities! When the body is stressed, try echinacea for a boost. Great for treating sore throats during a cold, the cold itself, flu symptoms, sore tissue and mild infections. Echinacea has antiseptic qualities and will aid in the treatment of septicaemia and other blood impurities. Many people who have cancer use this as a supplement (NOT replacement) to their treatments.
To make the tea steep the leaves, stem, flower and / or root of the plant in hot water for 10-15 minutes. The

infusion will bring out the polysaccharides and echinaceosides which contain the healthy stuff that echinacea has to offer.

Elder Flower Tea – Good for upper respiratory problems. Pour 1 cup boiling water over 2 teaspoons of dried elder flowers. Cover. Steep 3-5 minutes. Strain.

Elecampane Tea - Important note: Do NOT take if you are pregnant or nursing! *Large doses can cause vomiting, spasms, diarrhea and paralysis symptoms. Used as an expectorant to clear the lungs during bronchitis.
Pour 1 cup boiling water over 1 teaspoon of elecampane herb (dry). Cover. Steep 3-5 minutes. Strain.

Feverfew Tea - Important note: Do NOT use if pregnant. Do NOT use if youve had an allergic reaction to ragweed, daisies, chamomile, chrysanthemums or yarrow! Feverfew is a longtime remedy for many ailments. It contains wonderful nutrients including iron, niacin and Vitamins A and C. It is used in treating fever, arthritis, migraines, toothaches, psoriasis, menstrual cramping and possibly asthma. *If applied directly to the skin, it can be used as an insect repellent.

Put 1 teaspoon dry feverfew into 1 cup of water. Boil for 5-10 minutes. Strain the herbs out if not using an infuser ball.

Ginger Tea – Great for upset stomachs, motion sickness, gas, fresher breath and to aid in digestion. Put 1 teaspoon of ginger in 1 cup boiling water. Steep 5 minutes.

Ginkgo Biloba Tea -The leaves effect the lungs, kidneys and even increase circulation to the brain. The nuts of the ginkgo are an astringent and said to be a natural expectorant and sedative. May benefit asthmatics. Ginkgo contains flavonoids, glycosides, tannins and many other natural ingredients that are beneficial. Powerful antioxidants which seek out and slow down free radicals which contribute to dementia and premature aging. Used to improve mood, memory, concentration, tinnitus, circulation, vertigo, congestion in the chest, anxiety, tension and arthritis. Alzheimer patients and those suffering from senility may also see improvement.
Bring cold water to a rolling boil. Place ginkgo in an infuser ball, cover pot and steep for up to 8 minutes. (The longer, the stronger)

Ginseng Tea – Not used to cure things, but more of a boost when you are feeling ill. Make by steeping 5-7 slices of root, one teaspoon of powder or one tea bag for five -ten minutes depending on the strength desired. Ginseng mainly comes from Asia and is known for its stimulating abilities. There is a North American variety which is known more for its calming ability and is used for endurance and stamina. Ginseng is touted to have many health benefits including a stress reliever, immune strengthen, inflammation reducer including sore throats. The Chinese have used Ginseng for over 5,000 years!

Goldenseal Tea - Important note: Goldenseal may raise blood pressure. Should NOT be used by pregnant women or people with heart conditions.
Active constituents include: hydrastine, berberine, berberastine, canadine, candaline, hydrastinine, fatty acids, polyphenolic acids, resins, meconin, chlorogenic acid, phytosterins and tiny amounts of volatile oil. In order to get all the constituents released from the goldenseal, you must infuse the dry root or powder in boiling water for 5-10 minutes.
Benefits of goldenseal are: detoxifying on the whole body, helps diarrhea, relieves yeast infections, intestinal infections, respiratory infections, relief in eye diseases,

liver problems in alcoholics, and possibly in digesting fats.

Hawthorne Leaf / FlowerTea - Good for strengthening the heart and increasing blood flow. Pour 1 cup boiling water over 1 teaspoon of hawthorne leaves / flowers. Cover. Steep 3-5 minutes. Strain.

Hibiscus Tea - Has many antioxidants that protect the body from free radicals that damage cells. May help to control high blood pressure, high cholesterol and blood pressure. Since it has a high Vitamin C content it strengthens the immune system.
For tea: Pour 1 cup boiling water over 1 teaspoon dried (or 1 Tablespoon fresh) herb. Steep 3-8 minutes. Taste=Tangy, citrus

Horehound Tea – Important note: Do NOT use during pregnancy!
Good to fight severe congestion. Helps to make mucus and calms the bronchial muscles.
Pour 1 cup boiling water over 1/2 teaspoon of dry horehound herb. Cover. Steep 3-5 minutes. Strain.

Hyssop Tea - Important note: Do NOT use during pregnancy! Useful on sore throats.

Pour 1 cup boiling water over 1 teaspoon of dry hyssop. Cover. Steep 3-5 minutes. Strain.

Jasmine Tea – Not a true herbal tea but rather a real tea! Its green tea leaves and jasmine flowers.
Pour 1 cup boiling water over 1/4 teaspoon of dry jasmine flowers. Cover. Steep 3-5 minutes. Strain.

Juniper Berry Tea – Important note: Do NOT take if you are pregnant! Also, do not use for longer than 4 weeks in succession. Do NOT use if you have inflammatory kidney disease.
Pick in the autumn three years after the berries are formed.
Pour 1 cup boiling water over 1/2 teaspoon of dry juniper berries. Cover. Steep 3-5 minutes. Strain.

Kava-Kava Tea – It is said that this herb improves your overall health, mainly a healthy heart. Also said to lower cholesterol and balance out your blood pressure.

Lavender Tea- Calms the nerves and the mind. Relaxes muscles. May benefit headaches an open nasal passages.

Lemon Balm- Memory enhancer, relaxing, calming, clears the head/sharpens the mind. Great for students taking exams. Said to also help headaches, migraines, bloating, gas, digestion, upset stomach, ulcers, colds, flu, insomnia, uterine pain, menstrual cramps, diabetes, arthritis, mood swings, nervous heart, shingles, heart palpitations, candida, cancer, and may stimulate the thyroid, gallbladder, liver, kidneys, spleen and pancreas.

Put 1 teaspoon of crushed lemon balm 1 cup boiling water. Steep 10 minutes. Take only twice daily.

Lemongrass Tea – Important note: Do NOT use during pregnancy. Used for calming and lifting your spirits. Pour 1 cup boiling water over 1 teaspoon dried lemongrass herb. Cover. Steep 3-5 minutes.

Licorice Tea – Used by both eastern and western herbalists and for thousands of years. Called the elixir of life. The earliest clay Mesopotamian tablets ever found say that licorice was used as a panacea! The pharaohs in Egypt regularly drank licorice drinks!

Soothes a cough and sore throat. Said to improve digestion, wheezing, insomnia, anxiety, skin allergies, tension, candida, age spots, toothache, congestion, diabetes, gastritis, earache, headache, shingles, herpes, hormonal imbalances, chronic fatigue, high blood pressure, stomach ulcers, psoriasis, poor circulation, and relieve menstrual cramping. Studies are being conducted using licorice root as an ointment in the treatment of eczema, as well as many other uses involving licorice.

Rich in vitamins A, B1-2-5-6 & 9, and E. Rich in minerals too! Calcium, iron, magnesium, manganese, phosphorus, potassium, sodium, cobalt and zinc (among others). Contains: volatile oils, linolenic acid, alkaloids, tannins, phenols, flavonoids, salicylic acid, glycyrrhizin, mucilage, lecithin and protein and many more!

1 teaspoon licorice root or powder into 1 cup boiling water. Steep 10 minutes. Strain if using root. Can use 2x daily. *Not prolonged or excessive use which may cause depleted potassium and sodium retention. Can cause hypertension, headache, vertigo and edema. *Do NOT use if you have hypertension, hypokalemia, edema, cirrhosis of the liver, cholestatic liver or diabetes.

Lobelias Tea – Powerful when used against respiratory infections, to calm lymph nodes and earache and said to relieve symptoms of mono.

Masala Tea is a wonderful Indian beverage. Many of us call this a chai tea. Indians love this tea at any time of the day or night and understand its benefits. Tea refreshes the soul, lifts the spirit and helps the cells in our body regenerate. There is not really a set recipe for Masala Tea. Actually it varies somewhat in different cultures and in different regions. Whichever recipe you make, you will surely find this relaxing and refreshing. In some regions they use mint. In others, almonds. There are probably thousands of variations on this wonderful drink!

Here is a list of the basic Indian Masala chai tea ingredients: (can be found at most grocery stores)

* strong loose-leaf black tea such as Orange Pekoe or Assam
* cardamom (this is the predominant ingredient)
* ginger (second most predominant ingredient)
* cinnamon
* star anise or *cloves
* peppercorns

You can also purchase a powdered form of Masala Chai Tea. In this case you would just add it to the tea (or tea leaves), water and milk. Look for Indian tea brands such as Godrej, Double Diamond and Red Label (and there are many, many more).

*Note: Although sometimes you can buy this tea in bags that can be steeped you will lose much of the flavor. So why not take a few minutes and make it from scratch? Or, you can grind the dry ingredients and store it for a short time - using a teaspoon or two when you decide you want a cup. Just add the teaspoon or two to your black tea and add milk and sugar to taste.

Here is my favorite recipe!
* 3-4 Tablespoons loose orange pekoe tea (note, orange peoke doesn't mean it tastes like orange. It doesn't)
* 1 piece of dry ginger or 1/4 teaspoon crushed or ground
* 3 cardamom pods, crushed up
* 2 whole cloves
* 1/8 teaspoon ground peppercorn
* 1-2 cinnamon sticks (break in pieces)
*3 cups water
*1/2 cup milk
*sugar 1-2 tablespoons brown or white (you can always add a little more. You cannot take it away though)
Put the dry spices above into the 3 cups water and bring to a boil. Remove the pan from the heat, cover and steep 5 minutes. Add the 1/2 cup milk and sugar to the pan and bring to a boil again. Remove from the heat

and add the tea. Cover and let steep for 3 minutes. Stir the chai mixture and strain through a strainer or mesh material right into your cups.

Nettle Tea - Note: Nettles are often called stinging nettles because, of course, they are prickly and feel like they sting. Use caution when handling fresh nettles! Very high in Vitamins A and C. May clean the blood and improve kidney and liver function.

For tea: Can use the leaves and stem. Soak 1/2 cup (loosely packed) fresh nettles in cold water a few minutes. Separately, boil a pot of water (not with the nettles). Rinse cold nettles off, put into a cup, pour your boiling water over the nettles, and steep 5 minutes. Strain and drink.

Parsley Tea - Important note: Do NOT use during pregnancy! Do NOT use if you have inflammatory kidney disease! Said to improve kidney function, ease aches/pains.

Pour 1 cup boiling water over 1 teaspoon dry herb OR 2 teaspoons fresh parsley leaves (bruised with a spoon first) Cover and steep 10 minutes. Can drink 3x daily.

Peppermint Leaf Tea - Steep 1 Tablespoon in one cup boiling water for 3-5 minutes. Great for head colds, headaches, bronchitis, fever, stomach aches, digestive issues and stress relief. (And makes your breath fresh!)

Rooibos (roy-boss) or Red Tea - (contains oligosaccharides, a sugar compound that may help the immune system fight infections that are viral) Rooibosis high in antioxidants. Although there is no scientific evidence to support these theories, it is said that Rooibosteas may be beneficial for those suffering from hay fever and asthma, insomnia, tension, constipation, stomach cramping, eczema, acne and diaper rashes. Researchers have, however, found that Rooiboscontains a little fluoride, calcium and manganese as well as a flavonoidknown as Aspalathin which can be a treatment for skin or circulatory disorders. Made by putting leaves in the bottom of a cup and pouring hot water over them. Let sit 10 minutes. Drink hot or cold, with or without milk or cream.

Rose Hip Tea -After the petals fall off the rose, what is left is the fruit of the rose, or the rose hip. An excellent source of Vitamin C. (Sixty times the Vitamin C of citrus fruit and rose hips also have the bioflavonoids which aid absorbing Vitamin C.) Put a handful of hips (fresh or dry) into a cup of boiling water.

Let sit 10 minutes. Will be tart tasting, but good for colds and flu.

Rosemary Tea – Said to improve circulation, ease joint pain, relieve headache and stimulate the liver.
For sun-brewed tea: Place 6 tea bags (or 2 Tablespoons loose tea in an infuser ball) into a large pitcher with 1 1/2 quarts of cold water. Add 3-4 rosemary sprigs (lightly beaten with a spoon first). Add 3 lemon slices if desired. Put in the sun or indoors for 3 hours. Strain and remove tea bags/infuser ball.

Sage - Important note: Do NOT take if you are pregnant! Memory enhancer, calms the nerves, helps ease coughs and congestion in the chest, improves digestion.
1 Tablespoon fresh sage leaves or 1 teaspoon dried sage into 1 cup boiling water. Let steep 30 minutes. Flavor with honey, sugar or lemon if desired.

Sarsaparilla - For energy and healthy skin. Steep 2 teaspoons in 1 cup boiling water for 3 minutes. (More than a flavoring for root-beer, sarsaparilla has been used worldwide for thousands of years)

Skullcap Tea - Said to calm the nerves and reduce anxiety.
Steep 1/2 oz. powdered skullcap in 2 cups boiling water for 10 minutes. Only drink 4 ounces at a time, every few hours.

Slippery Elm - Used widely by Native Americans and pioneers internally for food, medicinally for kidney problems, dysentery, esophagitis, sore throat, bronchitis, diarrhea, constipation, stomach cramps and other gastrointestinal issues. Externally for such things as burns, chapped lips, wounds and skin problems.
For tea: 2 teaspoons ground slippery elm powder in 1 cup boiling water. Let sit 5 minutes. Can also be mixed into juice, pureed fruit, oatmeal, applesauce or other foods to soothe the stomach.

Spearmint Tea - Helps stomach aches, nausea, indigestion and heartburn. Great for morning sickness! Rinse spearmint leaves under cold water. Pour a cup of boiling water over 1 heaping teaspoon of spearmint tea leaves. Cover and steep for 2-5 minutes.

St. Johns Wort Tea -Important notes: Do NOT use during pregnancy, while taking anti-depressants, while taking over the counter cold/flu meds, when drinking alcohol, or when eating foods containing tyramine. *If you have high blood pressure, consult your doctor! *Do NOT take if you are also taking amino acid supplements!

Lifts the spirits, calming, relieves anxiety and crankiness. Said to help depression. St. Johns Wort contains hypericin which inhibits a chemical in the body that is associated with depression. The hypericincombined with other constituents in wort are what is said to help depression.

For tea: 1-2 cups flowers of St. Johns Wort to 1 cup of boiling water. Steep 10 minutes and strain. Can take 3x daily.

Thyme Tea - Good for bronchitis, sinusitis and whooping cough. Said to aid in digestion.

1 heaping teaspoon thyme to 1 cup boiling water. Steep 10 minutes. Strain if not using an infuser ball. *Do not exceed 3 cups daily.

Uva Ursi (see Bearberry)

Valerian Tea - Taken for relaxation because it's said to ease the nerves. Also touted as relief for stomach cramping, lowering blood pressure, relieving headaches, insomnia and anxiety. *Can be addictive and habit forming. **When making tea: Don't use hot water as it will deplete the active properties. Pour 1 cup of COLD water over 1 (level) teaspoon of chopped valerian root. Let sit overnight. When you are ready to drink it, you can warm it a bit if desired. Also, drinking a cup of valerian tea 45 minutes before bedtime will induce sleep. (And putting it into a bath will lift your spirits with its aroma)

White Peony Tea -Contains caffeine because it is actually a real tea taken from the camellia sinensis bush. The tea is harvested in the spring in China. White tea comes from the unopened bud of the plant. The white peony in the name comes from the steeping process where as the green leaves unfold and resemble the petals of a peony blossom. Sometimes this white tea is blended with daffodil plant. (There are no peony flowers in this tea). It is good for the stomach as well as all the benefits of real tea!

Use 2 heaping teaspoons per 6-7 ounces of boiling water. Steep 3 minutes. Strain if not using an infuser ball.

Yarrow Tea - Important note: Do NOT use during pregnancy or nursing. Do NOT use if you are allergic to ragweed, or if you have severe liver or kidney disease.

It is said that yarrow is useful in treating fevers because it makes you sweat. Also useful in fighting colds, flu, gas, gastritis, enteritis, stomach aches, helps poor circulation and helps calm inflammation. Also said to encourage menstruation and help overall functioning of the gallbladder.

Yarrow has tannins among many other constituents that give it the effect of a diaphoretic. This means that it causes surface capillaries and helps with circulation in the body.

Steep 1-2 Tablespoons of dried yarrow herb in 1 Cup of boiling water. Strain.

Yerba Mate Tea -The drink of the gods, Yerba Mate is actually a small tree grown in Argentina, Brazil and Paraguay. The tea is made from the dried leaves and stems. They say Yerba Mate has almost 200 volatile chemical compounds. It contains tannins, antioxidants, flavonoids, vitamins, amino acids, polyphenolsand saponins and all the nutrients to sustain life. It's also a diuretic, it breaks down glycogen in the liver, makes the heart beat stronger and faster, stimulates the nervous system and it breaks down fat. Yerba Mate also helps headaches, gastrointestinal issues and fatigue. It increases energy levels, clears your mind and even gifts metabolism a boost!

Modern methods of making this tea include using a coffee maker to brew it, a french press or with a tea infuser packed with dry leaves (2-4 minutes steeped). Add lemon, mint or sugar to hide the natural taste. Good cold and hot. You can also substitute milk for water when brewing.

Note: First place dry leaves in a cup and add cold water to moisten them. Then pour hot water in until all the leaves are covered. Leave the leaves in the bottom and drink through a straw.

Traditionally a cup of tea was shared as a sign of bonding and friendship. The host prepares the tea and drinks the first cup (the first cup is the strongest of the batch), makes adjustments to the taste, refills the cup and passes it to the next person who then drinks, passes it back to the host and the process repeats until all have had a cup. (But I'm a germ-a-phobe, therefore I don't recommend sharing.)

About the Author

Sheila Burke was born and raised in Northeast Ohio. In 1989 she married her soul mate Shane, and together they have delighted in raising their three beautiful children into strong young adults.

Always a dabbler in putting pen to paper, Burke finally started publishing her books in 2010 with the release of her first book Zen-Sational Living. Her journey of self-discovery started after getting over the hurdle of raising teenagers without losing all of her marbles. Learning how to live a life where stress takes a backseat and love rides shotgun is reflected in her writing. She shares her knowledge of spirit and soul, of all she understands, freely and simply through her many titles.

Other Books by Sheila Burke (available in bookstores)

Chorus of Souls: The Sacred Guide to Harmony, Healing, and Happiness (Jan 2014) Amazon **http://bit.ly/ChorusOfSouls**

"It is not the Universe conspiring against you - it is the Universe conspiring with you"

Our soul (our pure consciousness) is like the chorus of a song. It is the most powerful area of our structure, repeating itself over and over again. Not unlike the chorus of a song, the soul consciousness carries our message and expresses our main theme in the life we are here to live.

CHORUS OF SOULS is a guide for cultivating a healthy spiritual practice, a guide to a harmonious and happy life, and a guide to heal a sick soul. We all have the tools within ourselves to heal our soul and to live life in harmony and happiness.

Chorus of Souls delves into many areas including the actual benefits of meditation and prayer, arriving and departing souls, vibrational energy, how to forgive and the importance of forgiving, how we are all connected, and many more topics to nourish, strengthen, and heal your soul.

Transforming sacred and ancient knowledge into a clear and concise road map for the reader, Burke will inspire you to think, speak, and live authentically. Reacquaint yourself with your spirit through CHORUS OF SOULS.

Zen-Sational Living: A Simple Guide to Finding Your True Self and Maintaining Balance

Loaded with sensible advice, Zen-Sational Living is a road-map for making good decisions and being your best. From the basics of Zen, to health (mental and physical), creating a personal space, and everything in between! Whether you're in need of a boost, a change, or are starting on your own road of self-discovery, ZEN-SATIONAL LIVING will guide you on your journey. With easy to follow chapters on judgment, focus, compassion, forgiveness, stress, relaxation, and many more; Burke guides the reader in making simple, mindful adjustments for a healthier spirit, mind, and body. This book is truly an amazing guide on how to appreciate life and enjoy life.

Booyah! Spirit: 52 Ingredients for a Healthy Soul. Suffering Is Optional

BOOYAH! SPIRIT merges scientific research, humor, wonderful pictures, quotes, how-tos, and personal life lessons to help you live the life of your dreams. The expression "Booyah" is one that many people would yell after one performs a difficult feat. But I also discovered that Booyah "is a food that is prepared like a stew, but on a very large scale. It takes many cooks to prepare the food, and it is usually meant to serve hundreds or even thousands of people". Not unlike Booyah Stew, this book is filled with ideas to nourish the souls of hundreds or even thousands of people. BOOYAH! SPIRIT combines ancient ideas with new ones. There are 52 chapters that represent the weeks of the year.

Circle of Soul: at the end, we begin again

CIRCLE OF SOUL guides the reader through finding their inner Spirit - a place that for many has become lost over time through the rigors of everyday life. Sages throughout the ages have taught us how to live a spiritual life - it is not a secret. A personal journey doesn't have to be difficult, this book will help you get started and on your way.

Whispers of the Soul

WHISPERS OF THE SOUL is the 5th title released by inspirational author Sheila M. Burke. Whispers is a full color poster book filled with the author's original photography and original quotes about the soul, soul mates, and soul connections.

Did you ever meet someone and become fast friends, where you feel as if you have known them your entire life, although you've only just met recently? I know those feelings well; I have them on occasion. I think they are leftover energies, imprints if you will, left upon the universe from times past. A wink and smile and perhaps a bond from another time that went deep. Coming full circle and finding you again in this lifetime.

150 Ways to Get Your Zen On: Book 1 – Finding Your Happy Place

150 Ways to Get Your Zen On: Book 2 – Simple Pleasures

It's the simple things we do or enjoy daily that help us find our Zen. Belly laughs, the warmth of a sunrise, kindness, puppy kisses, or thick, fuzzy socks. The little things that help you to relax and let all the stress slide off your shoulders.

These books provide 150 examples each of simple thinking designed to help you find your happy place. Zen is not about never feeling sad, angry, joyful, or having fun; Zen is the understanding that by not clinging (or attaching) ourselves to these feelings, we can free ourselves from them and enjoy life to the fullest.

www.sheilamburke.com
(Portal to all offerings! ZenSational Living, Irie, Photos, Courses, Books, and my Facebook Pages for ZenSational and Irie! Join me there!) www.sheilamburke.com/courses (Join our eCourses!)

Irie is like Namaste, but with an island flavor! A fun inspirational place for those seeking and sharing happiness, harmony, and appreciation for life.

ZenSational Living is about the simple life, spirit, and soul.

www.ingramcontent.com/pod-product-compliance
Lightning Source LLC
Chambersburg PA
CBHW070119290526
45789CB00005B/2067